Yoga for Beginners

A Complete Guide on Yoga Poses for Beginners

Stacy Milescu

GW00770976

This book is dedicated to anyone looking to achieve strength, flexibility, weight loss, better overall health or inner peace through the practice of yoga.

Speedy Publishing LLC (c) 2014
40 E. Main St., #1156
Newark, DE 19711
www.speedypublishing.co

Ordering Information:
Quantity sales; Special discounts are available on quantity purchases by corporations, associations, and others. For details, contact the "Special Sales Department" at the address above.

-- 1st edition

Manufactured in the United States of America

TABLE OF CONTENTS

PUBLISHER'S NOTES

Disclaimer

This publication is intended to provide helpful and informative material. It is not intended to diagnose, treat, cure, or prevent any health problem or condition, nor is intended to replace the advice of a physician. No action should be taken solely on the contents of this book. Always consult your physician or qualified health-care professional on any matters regarding your health and before adopting any suggestions in this book or drawing inferences from it.

The author and publisher specifically disclaim all responsibility for any liability, loss or risk, personal or otherwise, which is incurred as a consequence, directly or indirectly, from the use or application of any contents of this book.

Any and all product names referenced within this book are the trademarks of their respective owners. None of these owners have sponsored, authorized, endorsed, or approved this book.

Always read all information provided by the manufacturers' product labels before using their products. The author and publisher are not responsible for claims made by manufacturers.

Print Edition 2014

CHAPTER 1: WHAT IS YOGA AND HOW DID IT START?

Yoga is a word that you have probably heard of before, but you might not know what it actually means. The word itself, Yoga, is described as meaning "to join" or "to yoke together." This is because the practice of Yoga is intended to bring both the mind and the body together to form and behave, as a single harmonious existence.

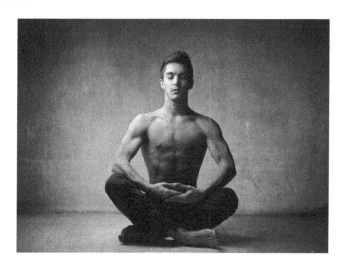

Yoga has been around for so very long now, that its true origin has become lost through the ages of time. Some practitioners are of the belief that it could be as ancient as 10,000 years old. This is because much of the knowledge surrounding Yoga was passed on verbally, instead of through books. This let knowledge be forgotten through time, including the date of Yoga's exact origins.

However, in Pakistan, there have recently been figures that were unearthed during archaeological exhibitions in the Indus Valley.

Seals carved out of soapstone were unearthed with some surprising imagery on them. These seals, which were located in the Mohenjo-Daro dig site, were from the Indo-Saraswati people and each had a figure depicted upon them that was in various Yoga poses.

These stone seals can be dated back to 3,000 B.C. That is over 5,000 years ago! Because this is the oldest physical evidence, the true age of the origins of Yoga itself are suspected to go back much further to a time before documenting onto the carvings existed. If the past was anything like the present, then we know that something has to first be popular before it becomes documented for others to attempt it. Yoga could be as old as 26,000 years according to some archaeologists who have been studying its origins. Interestingly, one of the world's oldest text known as the Rig-Veda; which is a composition of hymns, is known to contain evidence of Yoga mentioned within its tomes.

Amazingly, they are identifiable. One of the figures that was discovered on the soapstone carvings is without a doubt a figure depicting that of the God Shiva, who is known as the God of Yoga. There are many attributes that support this belief, ranging from the image having three faces, to the crown of buffalo horns depicted on the seal, all known items associated with the God Shiva.

When it comes down to putting a name to the teachings behind Yoga as we know it today, then you might be interested in hearing about Patanjali. There are many people who believe that a philosopher named Patanjali is the true father of Yoga. This is because during the ancient times, Yoga poses and their techniques were not transcribed into manuals for students to learn from. Instead of manuals or posters designed to illustrate the movements, Yoga instead was taught from the teacher to their students, directly. It is believed that 2,000 years ago, Patanjali made the effort to create a documented collection of organized principles into a compilation known as Yoga Sutras. This made it easier to teach and distribute the principals of Yoga to more people across the globe.

There are essentially 3 structures that Yoga is built upon: meditation, exercise and breathing.

The sound, Aum; which is often spelled "Om," is an important aspect of the practice of Yoga. The sound is considered vital, because it is thought to be the one sound that connects the entire universe. The one word is represented as three sounds for destruction, creation and preservation. The sound, or word, is chanted often during meditations or closing of prayer during Yoga practice. It is believed that the whole of speech and thought come from one source, the sound aum.

It is further thought, that to chant the sound aum, creates a feeling of sacredness. That to achieve true understanding of the sound, it must be heard from inside of yourself, spreading out to become one with it and in so doing, becoming one with creation. It does not matter if the sound is uttered aloud, whispered under the breath or if it is only heard mentally. What matters is that the sound, "aum," is uttered correctly to sound as if it rhymes with the word "home."

The recommended technique is to begin with "aum" being repeated for upwards of ten minutes out loud. Following this, repeat the chant but using only a whisper for the same duration of time. When done, repeat a final time but only within your mind are you to chant the sound, also for ten minutes. Now is when it is recommended to begin meditating on your spiritual eye. The spiritual eye is non-tangible and is thought to be located between the eyebrows. Allow yourself to sense the vibrations of the sound "aum" with the desire to expand your awareness until you are one with the very sound itself. This is the sensation that many Yoga practitioners strive to attain.

3

Yoga is somewhat new to the U.S. It was first reported being practiced in the United States back in the 1890's. Widespread attention and acceptance of the practice was not seen, however, until the 1960's.

Due to its popularity, Yoga has been found in many Eastern religions from Hinduism, Hari Krishna, Jainism and Sikhism. Some Christian organizations have also incorporated Yoga practice into the prayer and meditation. The latter has been of hot debate with some who take offense that a Hindu-based spiritual principal would be overcast with Christian ideology.

If you are considering the practice of Yoga, it is advised that you try and attend a free class or two, to see which instructor is offering what you need. If this is not an option then it is recommended that you speak to current members of classes that interest you to see if they would recommend it to another. You may find that there are numerous exercise classes that offer Yoga that is only exercises and stretching without any focus on the spiritual, body-mind connection, while others incorporate a deep spirituality.

CHAPTER 2: WHAT ARE THE ADVANTAGES OF PRACTICING YOGA?

Yoga practitioners often speak of the numerous benefits that are obtained from the correct postures and breathing that is associated with Yoga. If you suffer from a stressful life, such as a hectic work environment, then you might want to consider taking up Yoga. Yoga takes advantage of breathing techniques which require that you inhale and exhale during your movements.

These techniques can relieve tension that tends to build up in the body. Energy has been known to dramatically increase from repeated use of Yoga techniques. People have reported feeling refreshed and energized throughout even the most demanding of days. Even when exposed to only a few minutes of Yoga on a daily basis, practitioners were able to use guided meditation to feel recharged and new.

Yoga will build muscle tone while maintaining a correctly balanced metabolism. This is great for helping to regulate your weight. Cellulite is commonly reduced, due to how yoga postures stretch your muscles lengthwise, which destroys the fat around cells. While performing Yogic poses you will be required to focus on your breathing. This is very helpful in reducing stress and anxiety. Yogic breathing can be utilized almost anywhere; your car, office, or even in an elevator, to help maintain calm. Yoga includes a practice known as pranayama, and it's a breathing practice that has been shown to be effective at stress reduction. Lung function is also noted to have been improved while deeply encouraging relaxation. Through the use of alternating breathing styles, the body's experience of how to respond to stress can be better controlled.

5

The practice of reducing and deepening the breath is known to stimulate one's relaxation response over time.

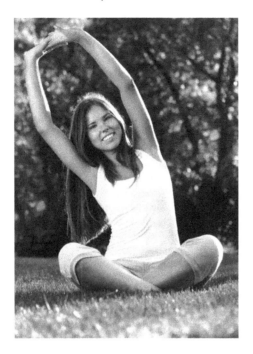

Your body will become well-toned while becoming flexible and strong. Respiration is improved along with vitality and athletic performance. Yoga is often useful for supporting weight loss. Even the most gentle of Yoga practices is known to support weight loss. Yoga practice highly encourages the formation of a positive self-image while focusing on nutrition and the body as a unit. Losing weight is possible even with the most minimal practicing of Yoga techniques. A recent study came to the conclusion that frequent practice of Yoga techniques had a direct correlation to a reduction in age-related weight gain. Obesity can easily be managed through Yoga classes practiced for 90-minutes, between 3 and 5 times a week.

You might even notice that pain has become greatly reduced, while overall, you will look and feel younger. Research determined that

Yoga postures combined with meditation was highly effective at reducing chronic pain associated with arthritis, cancer, auto-immune diseases, multiple sclerosis, back pain and more.

Yoga will greatly improve circulation because it quiet effectively transports oxygen rich blood to your body's cells. Research has proven that even the most minimal amount of time spent practicing Yoga will lower your resting heart rate, improve endurance and advance oxygen uptake. Better sleep can be attained if you are among one of the millions of Americans who is currently suffering from insomnia. Frequent practicing of Yoga has been known to have a substantial impact on helping to obtain a better night's sleep. Yoga can also encourage better posture through strengthening your core, within on a few weeks of Yoga techniques. Walking with confidence will come with newfound ease due to you frequent use of correct posture through Yoga.

Continued practice of Yoga aids with memory and concentration, and has been proven in recent studies to help prevent Alzheimer's disease. Yoga is known to be low impact, so there is no concern if you experience joint trouble or are elderly. It is strenuous to perform, however, so it is advised that you seek your doctor's advice before performing any exercise. You will also notice that muscle tone becomes defined while your weight becomes a more healthy and attractive silhouette. As a stress reliever, Yoga has long been known to be effective against stress if practiced often. Clearing your mind on a regular basis while you maintain focus on your body and your breathing can greatly diminish your reactions to stress.

An awareness of your body can be developed through Yoga practice, which is useful for noticing your outer world and the needs of those around you. You can develop an interrelationship with your spirit, mind and body. Many feel this promotes an understanding of the concept of "oneness." Over time, exposure to the techniques of Yoga practice can create a heightened awareness of your surroundings. This can also lead to a degree of improved reaction time, memory and coordination. Many find Yoga to be relaxing, a place where the mind can be quiet, allowing energy to be directed where needed. Positive thoughts become encouraged through repetition. All religions have practitioners who also practice Yoga. Yoga has no actual denomination. The thought behind Yoga is learning how to live in harmony with ourselves as well as others.

You might notice that relationships improve from your friends, to your spouse and other loved ones. It is known that when the mind is calm and content, that we are better capable of handling personal, private or sensitive matters. Yoga practice through meditation can be a great service to keeping the mind peaceful. Interestingly, many practitioners of Yoga have experienced an increase of intuition allowing for a seamless awareness of what is required to achieve positive results.

Menopausal women were found to report a 30% decrease in hot flashes after partaking in a two month session of weekly Yoga practice. Another study discovered that a large number of women who participated in a 90-minute Iyengar class on a regular basis had a marked increase in energy, and they commented on a decrease in sexual and physical pain, stress and anxiety in general.

It is advised that caution be taken as there are specific positions of Yoga that might lead to back, neck, shoulder, hip or knee pain. If you have existing neck or back problems or a musculoskeletal problem, exercise with caution.

CHAPTER 3: DOES YOGA IMPROVE YOUR HEALTH?

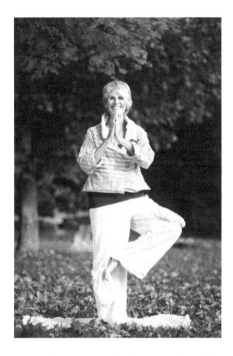

The art of yoga has been mainly designed to focus on the total wellness of an individual. When a person gets involved with yoga they will certainly learn new types of lifestyle ideas as well as new ways of approaching life within the world. Yoga has the ability to improve your health in numerous different ways.

Yoga has been shown to improve the health of those who practice it, in many ways. These include mental and physical health as well as, for some, spiritual aspects of their lives. Yoga can have dramatic effects on the lives of many people.

One area where that can be evident is in general blood circulation. Yoga exercises are very good for improving blood circulation and for anyone suffering from a circulatory problem it is well worth considering taking up Yoga, after a suitable consultation with your doctor. And blood circulation is important to so many aspects of our health.

All the tissues in our bodies need to move regularly to function properly. Witness what happens to those who are bedridden and suffer all sorts of problems related to their inability to move around enough.

The practice of Yoga ensures a good flow of blood to the tissues of our body. This in turn ensures a supply of oxygen because blood carries oxygen. And this helps improve the functioning of our organs and our general health. It will help in many areas of our general physical and mental health.

Those who suffer from mental problems such as reduced memory may well also find that the regular practice of Yoga and the resultant improvement in oxygen supply to the brain from improved blood circulation results in some improvement to their specific mental problems.

This can be true in so many areas of our lives. Yoga can be beneficial during pregnancy for example, and there are many women who suffer from circulatory problems during pregnancy. The practice of Yoga can help maintain the woman's overall health and mental well being and this may well in turn give her better physical ability and confidence to help her with the delivery.

There are all sorts of other physical conditions which can be improved with improved blood circulation which results from the practice of Yoga. Perhaps you will find that blood pressure problems improve, or back pain may improve or even just that you get a better night's sleep.

There are many benefits to be found from a disciplined practice of Yoga, many stemming from improvements in the overall circulatory function. There are even some particular Yoga exercises called Inversions which are especially developed to improve stamina and the strength of the upper body, and these also help improve blood circulation.

Inversions keep your legs above the level of your heart which in turn affects the flow of blood. They should be done after long periods of standing. There are some who should avoid inversions, such as pregnant women, and anyone suffering from a specific medical problem should of course consult their doctor first.

Yoga is a discipline like any other, and so the benefits you get from it will depend on the degree to which you practice Yoga, however if you do so regularly, don't be surprised to find your overall health increasing.

There are many Yoga poses that can improve overall health by improving the circulation. Consult your instructor if you'd like to learn more about the effects of Yoga on circulation, and find out more about the specific Yoga exercises to help you improve your circulation.

There are a range of health benefits from the practice of Yoga. These range from improvements in general levels of health and fitness, to improvements in mental health in some cases, and to, for some, an expansion of what could best be described as spiritual health. Yoga has wide ranging benefits.

Yoga can lessen stress in your life, and help with some problems such as anxiety. And one area where the disciplined practice of Yoga helps greatly is flexibility. The regular practice of Yoga can make a big difference to your flexibility.

Yoga is a low impact, slow and invigorating form of stretching exercise. It is not specifically designed with stretching in mind, but this is certainly one of it's benefits. As Yoga exercises or movements are done slowly and carefully, over time this will lead to an improvement in your overall flexibility and this will make differences in other areas of your life.

Improvements in flexibility can reduce muscle strain from trying to do things which your current flexibility prohibits without effort. It can improve back movement and muscle pain and will sometimes help with such problems as migraines.

Simple things like sitting at your office desk or reaching to pick something up may be more comfortable. Bending over will become easier. You may well find that other activities, particularly sporting and recreational activities become more enjoyable as your flexibility improves.

These are just a few of the benefits of Yoga. Yoga is easy to learn, although it does take some discipline to do it regularly, as with many forms of exercise. It can be practiced by people with no experience and is easy to take bit by bit. There is no requirement to do a certain amount, you can take it at your own pace and learn as slow or as fast as you like.

When you learn Yoga at your pace it has limited risk of injury as it is a slow low impact form of exercise. Yoga is fun and healthy. If you're thinking of taking up Yoga give it a go. You won't regret it.

Yoga is great for completely messaging your internal organs as well as the glands of your upper body which includes those that infrequently get the stimulation needed. Through the use of messaging your organs as well as your glands yoga assists your bodies defenses to resist diseases from harming your health.

A substantial benefit of doing yoga is the added blood flow that happens throughout your physical body which adds to the strength of your health. The added flow of blood substantially helps your body's natural ability to lower toxin substances as well as delivers added nourishments through your body.

CHAPTER 4: DISCOVER THE DIFFERENT TYPES OF YOGA

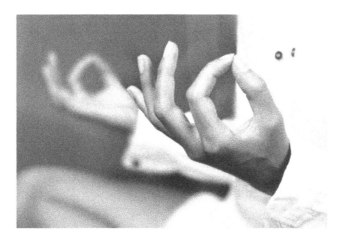

Deciding that you want to take part in yoga is great, but it can get a little confusing when you learn that there is more than one type. In order to narrow down your selection, you need to be objective about your current physical fitness and where you would like to end up physically and spiritually.

Each yoga type is defined by a specific set of functions and characteristics that are targeted towards an approach to life. There are some that you are sure to love, and others not so much. Just keep in mind that when you settle on one type of yoga, it does not mean that you have to shun the others, as some of the techniques will in fact overlap.

Listed below are some of the most common forms of yoga and a brief explanation of what you can expect from each. This should help you choose the best one for you.

Iyengar Yoga – Your focus here will be on inner awareness, alignment, and precise movements. For the awareness aspect, you need to start with your body and slowly expand outwards as you practice regularly.

Props are often used to help make each pose be attained comfortably. Each of the poses is flexible to modification, which makes this type of yoga especially helpful to those who suffer from pain in the neck and back. The random alteration of poses is what helps those folks deal with their pain so effectively.

Ashtanga Yoga – The focus on powerful flowing movement is why this style is often referred to as power yoga. Strength and stamina are required to perform the lunges and push-ups that are featured here, making this a style that is definitely for those looking for more of a challenge. Block, straps, and other props are often employed in this type of yoga, especially if you are at the beginner level and perhaps not as flexible as is required.

This form of yoga is actually incredibly popular among athletes who rely on power and balance in the sport or activity that they take part in.

Bikram Yoga: This type of yoga is performed in a warm environment, which is why it is often referred to as hot yoga. It is commonly used to increase flexibility.

There is a word of warning that comes with this yoga type, and it is that it is not recommended for those with cardiovascular issues. The heat and strain on the body can become a major issue in those cases.

Tantra Yoga: There may be no more spiritual type of yoga than Tantra, with the literal meaning of the word being "expansion." Delving into Tantra means opening up one's consciousness on many levels so that the Supreme Reality can be reached. Both the male and female aspects are awoken in order to attain a true spiritual awakening.

Raja Yoga: This is considered by many to be one of the most difficult forms of yoga, with the goal to find freedom through meditation. In order to find enlightenment, you are required to control and master the mind, which is a tall order for most. The people best suited to Raja yoga are those who are able to meditate and give over to deep concentration.

Raja yoga splinters off into 8 separate limbs:

- Moral discipline
- Self-restraint
- Posture
- Breath control
- Sensory inhibition
- Concentration
- Meditation
- Ecstasy

Bhakti Yoga: This type of yoga asks you to surrender yourself in the face of the divine, which is why it is often referred to as the path of devotion. Through this type of yoga you will learn to become tolerant and accepting of everyone you encounter.

Mantra Yoga: This is more commonly referred to as the "yoga of potent sound," as you seek liberation via the use repeated sounds such as "om," "hum," and "ram."

CHAPTER 5: WHAT TO WEAR WHEN PRACTICING YOGA

Yoga is a wonderful way to get fit. There are various forms of yoga, from soft and relaxing types that focus on flexibility, to very intense forms of yoga that will have you redefine your ideas about what calisthenics can be. So now you're all hyped for yoga and have signed up for classes. What to wear though?

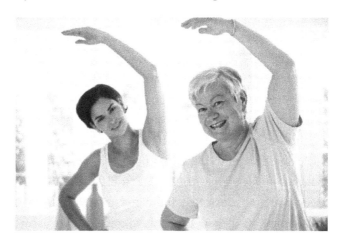

It's easiest to start off with what not to wear. Nothing constricting, you need to be flexible. Since you're going to be stretching into a variety of positions avoid clothing with zippers or buttons that could pinch your skin. For that same reason trimmed nails would be more comfortable. If you have long hair get it up and out of the way. Don't fuss with cute hairstyles, opt for comfort and practicality. An up do might look sweet and sophisticated but will easily get undone, especially if your poses have you laying your head flat on the ground. Avoid claw clips for that same reason; it isn't comfortable to lay down with a claw clip in your hair. Also try to avoid "swishy-sounding" materials that can be a distraction.

Many yoga instructors place a premium on relaxation and concentration so avoid any clothing or accessories that could make noise and distract fellow classmates. If you're signed up for high intensity yoga leave the makeup at home, you'll be sweating it all off anyway. Don't wear perfume or heavily scented lotions. Don't bother with sneakers or flip flops. Your feet will probably contort along with the rest of you so you want shoes that offer a bit more flexibility, if you want to wear any to begin with since you'll notice most of your classmates will be barefoot. Don't wear loose shorts. You'll be stretching and contorting every which way, you don't want to worry about anyone being able to see up your shorts (if you wear shorts they should be tight).

So now you know what to avoid; it might sound a little limiting but it is absolutely possible to be stylish and prepared for class. First up are yoga pants. What makes yoga pants different from any other kind of pants? Well they're flexible, comfortable, and the materials aren't as warm and suffocating as other kinds of fabrics. Yoga pants should breathe. You can even buy varieties that are made of special 'moisture-wicking' fabric, which could be a very welcome addition the wardrobe of anyone who sweats just a little too much. Before wearing your pants to class test them out in front of the mirror first. Many women have had the unfortunate embarrassment of wearing yoga pants that became only semi-opaque when stressed and stretched. You can buy yoga pants in many different cuts and lengths, but light colors are always more likely to be see through. There's a reason most yoga pants are black!

The classic conception of yoga pants is long and tight, but looser yoga pants exist and might be a good option for some people since they breathe a little bit better as the fabric isn't pressed up against the skin. You can also buy yoga shorts for the warmer months. Since yoga pants can fit very tight it is easy to have visible panty line showing through. Wear thinner underwear or thongs with your tighter yoga pants. Some underwear fabric retains heat and sweat more than others, so make sure you know which panties you find most comfortable. Men's yoga pants are often less form-fitting. Some pants might have little pockets, which would be handy for anyone that has to walk or bus home.

Your tops should be made of comfortable, breathable fabric. Many men practice yoga bare-chested and many women will wear only a sports bra. If you're wearing a sports bra make sure it is comfortable. Many women make the mistake of buying sports bras that aren't as supportive as their normal underwire bras. Yoga likely won't give a woman much trouble or pain in the way of 'bounce' but that's no reason to neglect a well-fitting sports bra. There are sports bras with underwire and others with individual cups, which can be especially comfortable.

Other sports bras have mesh panels to help skin breath just a bit more. Some women will find themselves more comfortable wearing a sports bra or camisole that has a little padding in the front for a smoother look. Women with bigger breasts should be especially wary of the thickness of the straps. Thinner straps may not bother a less busty woman but are less supportive for her larger-chested counterpart. "Racerbacks" might be more comfortable than regular straps since they distribute weight differently. Some bras have little inserts in which to place an mp3 player (only use them with ear buds!).

On top of you sports bra you can wear a cute camisole. Smaller breasted women can wear the camisole on with no bra underneath. Sports bras and camisoles come in a variety of colors and necklines; though in almost all cases sleeveless will be more comfortable. Feel free to experiment, mix and match different cuts and color of top and bottoms. Opt for a top that is fairly form-fitting. Some yoga poses practically have you upside down and you don't want the shirt to succumb to gravity, it can get annoying and you may end up baring more skin than you feel comfortable with.

Low cut tops may not be a good option for women with larger breasts, you don't want to feel like you're popping out of your shirt when you're doing the downward dog!

Other things you may consider bringing include headbands to soak up the sweat on your forehead, a towel to mop up your face with afterward, and clothing for getting back home. This is especially pertinent for anyone who will be walking to class. Class can be a short affair or it can last hours. The weather outside may have been comfortable when you first arrived but it might be chilly when you leave. Maybe you only need to pack a jacket, or maybe you'll need a full change of clothing.

CHAPTER 6: THE IMPORTANCE OF BREATHING TECHNIQUES WHEN PRACTICING YOGA

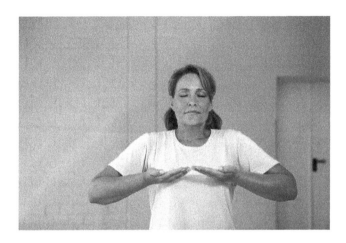

Proper breathing is a key element of yoga, because it nourishes every cell of the human body. Without a constant fresh supply of oxygen to each cell through respiration, our cells quickly become damaged and unable to perform, denying us the energy that they normally provide. Yoga teaches the correct way to inhale and exhale, so that we use each breath efficiently, avoiding the pitfalls that incorrect breathing creates. Amazingly, seventy percent of our body's waste materials are expelled through our lungs, according to The Tao of Natural Breathing by Dennis Lewis. Therefore, the art of breathing that is so crucial to yoga is given a special name - pranayama.

When we breathe oxygen into our lungs, it does not stop there, but instead mixes with hemoglobin to become oxyhemoglobin. This enables the oxygen to disperse throughout the body by way of our circulatory system. Blood carries oxygen to every tiny part of our body to nourish individual cells, which keeps us alive. Since yoga is all about being mindful of a healthy existence, it makes sense that a great emphasis is put on the most crucial piece of life-force, which is breathing.

Furthermore, breathing not only brings oxygen to our cells, it also takes away toxic substances like carbon dioxide from our system. Through a process called respiration, each time we breathe, oxygen-rich air is exchanged for air that contains carbon dioxide through diffusion. Deep breathing keeps this exchange of good air for bad moving smoothly while the entire air capacity of the lungs is refreshed. Moreover, deep thoughtful breaths can increase lung capacity, thereby helping people increase their abilities and endurance for sports.

Breathing is an automatic process that the body is hard-wired to carry out, whether we think about it or not. However, when we forget to practice deep breathing it is easy to fall into the trap of shallow breathing only. This causes us to use just the top one-third of our lung's capacity, which leaves the bottom two-thirds holding stagnant air. Meanwhile, the body's tissue, organs and fluids are deprived of the oxygen they must have to survive. This is why a human can only live an average of six minutes without breathing.

The human brain, however, needs more oxygen than any other organ in the body. Without the basic requirements of oxygen, sluggishness, bad thoughts and depression start to take over. Next, the individual's vision and hearing starts going downhill. The rest of the body begins losing its oxygen supply as people age, especially if they do not live a healthy lifestyle.

In addition, by breathing slower and deeper we can banish stress and impart a sense of peace and calmness in our self. These are essential goals when practicing yoga. Moreover, with every inhale and exhale the yoga practitioner can gain energy and create a stronger and deeper connection between mind and body. Generally, yoga teaches that as you breathe in, you gain more energy; inhaling is the best time to move while using, or contracting, the muscles. Alternately, exhaling is best for stretching and relaxing. Nevertheless, there are slight variations in breathing techniques between alternate styles of yoga.

Here are the four types of pranayama breathing techniques and why they are useful in yoga:

- Ujjayi pranayama - known as the victory breath, ujjayi is a way of breathing where the person makes a gentle hissing sound as they exhale due to the way that they direct the air over the back of their throat. Ujjayi is both relaxing and energizing, and it causes a slower rate of breathing that is uniform, which keeps the mind from wandering.

- Kapalabhati pranayama - this is the skull and sinuses cleansing breath, where the breather exerts more energy on the exhalation in order to fully expel all of the dead air in the bottom of the lungs. Inhaling comes naturally without putting any focus on it.

- Nadhi sodahana pranayama - here the emphasis is on breathing through one nostril at a time, in order to affect the opposite side of the brain. Known also as nostril breathing, the person holds one nostril closed by pressing it on the side, which allows the full breath of air to flow in and out through the other nostril. By breathing through the right nostril, the left side of the brain creates a sense of calmness. Alternately, breathing through the left nostril enhances the right side of the brain that is responsible for thinking skills.

- Sithali pranayama - this type of breathing cools the breather's body temperature when it becomes overheated. In addition, it is a moistening, uplifting and youthful breath, which works quickly in hot weather. First, the person must learn to curl, or roll, their tongue into a canal-like passageway that is open in the front. Next, they inhale air through this passageway with their mouth just slightly open. Exhaling takes place through the nose in a slow manner.

Hence, the importance of breathing certain ways during yoga is due to the calming, focusing effects as well as nourishing our cells while removing poisonous toxins from the body. Stress-reduction through calming yoga exercises, along with correct breathing techniques, can lengthen a person's lifetime while making it more enjoyable. Since people breathe an average of 24,000 times each day, there are many opportunities to renew and rejuvenate ourselves and create a healthy bond between our mind, body and soul.

By practicing controlled breathing through yoga, some of the negative conditions that may improve include chronic fatigue syndrome, chronic pain, depression, high blood pressure, asthma, insomnia and even certain skin problems like eczema. However, the largest improvements are in lowering anxiety levels, negative stress and panic attacks. Conversely, shallow chest breathing leads to eventual constriction of the chest and lung tissue, which decreases oxygen delivery to vital tissues and organs.

Many Eastern cultures realized long ago that how we breathe and move has a direct effect on our overall health. Yoga is a very healthy way of incorporating superior breathing, harmony and better health into our life. Ultimately, after all the positive effects of mindful deep breathing, there are no negative side effects to worry about and if does not cost money - anyone can enjoy the amazing benefits of breathing as taught through yoga.

CHAPTER 7: 15 BASIC YOGA POSES FOR BEGINNERS

Yoga is expressed by practicing a variety of poses. Before starting this or any other exercise program, consult a doctor, especially if you are pregnant.

Easy Pose: also known as Sukhasana. A basic and foundational pose that is great for beginners. This pose is seated with your legs criss crossed. Let your hands rest on top of your knees either palms up or down. Draw your chin to your chest, navel draws back and roll you shoulder and spine forward and inhale deeply. As you exhale rock your pelvis down and slowly roll back up towards an upright position.

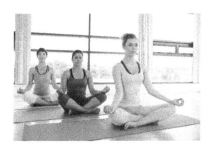

Mountain Pose: one of the easier poses to master. The Sanskrit name is Tadasana. To perform this pose, you will stand with feet at a hips distance apart. Your weight needs to be evenly spread. Place your arms at either side of your body. Slowly breathe at an even and deep pace while making certain that your neck is aligned with your spine. If you need to for focus, you can move your hands and arms. You might find some people who prefer to reach up towards the sky in a stretching or praying position.

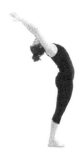

Tree Pose: also known as Vriksasana, is an evolution of the Mountain Pose. While in the Mountain Pose, alternate your weight onto your left leg while keeping your hips forward facing. The sole of your right foot should be placed onto the inside of your left thigh and be sure to find your balance. This is the point where you should transition into the prayer pose with your hands. You can also choose to stretch your arms up. Repeat these steps for the other side.

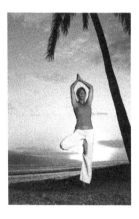

Warrior Pose: called Virabhadrasana in Sanskrit, is also performed while standing. Begin with your legs approximately four feet apart from one another. Now, turn your right foot outward 90 degrees. Your left foot should be turned slightly inward. Be certain to keep your shoulders down while extending your arms to your side. Keep your palms facing down and thrust into your right knee at 90 degrees. Do not let your knee go past the distance of your toes, but be sure that your knee is over your foot. Keep your focus directed over your hand until you feel like switching to the other side.

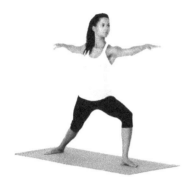

Triangle Pose: the English term for Trikonasana. Transition from the Warrior Pose on your right side but take care not to thrust into the knee. Take the outside of your right hand and use it to touch the inside of your right foot. Use your left hand, to reach up high towards the ceiling. Keep your eye line focused on your left hand as you stretch your back in this pose. Repeat this for the other side.

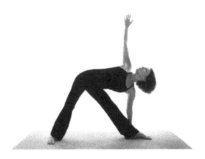

Downward Facing Dog: a popular pose. The Sanskrit name is Adho mukha svanasana. Begin by being on all fours, hands and knees should be set shoulder distance and hips width distance apart. Now, walk your hands forward and position your fingers spread eagle to maintain support. Press your hips forward until your body forms an inverted "V' shape while making sure that your knees are bent slightly and that your toes are curled under.

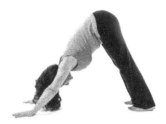

Crow Pose: also known as Bakasana, is a step beyond the Downward Dog Pose. From this position, walk your feet forward with the intent of touching your arms with your knees. Now, slowly bend your elbows while lifting your heels up from the floor. At this point, position your knees to the outside of your upper arms. Your abdomen muscles need to be tight and press your legs against your arms. It is ok to leave your toes on the floor. However, you can attempt to lift your toes and keep them afloat. To accomplish this, keep your rear tucked in tight with your heels near your rear. Now, push your upper arms into your shins while drawing your groin deeply into your pelvis and this will greatly assist you with your lifting.

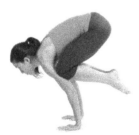

Upward Facing Dog: or Urdhva mukha svanasana, is performed from a floor position. While lying face down, position your thumbs beneath your shoulders. Be sure to extend your legs with the tops of your feet positioned against the floor. Now, tuck your hips down while contracting the muscles in your rear. Maintain your shoulders in a down position and push up while lifting your chest off the floor. Breathe and relax, and then repeat this maneuver.

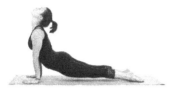

Bridge Pose: another pose that begins from the floor. In Sanskrit, it's called Setu bhanda. From a lying position on your back on the floor, place your arms out to your sides. Bend your knees and lift your hips while pressing your feet into the floor. Your hands should now clasp under your lower back. From here, press down with your arms to maintain stability. This is when you should lift up your hips to be parallel with the floor. Bring your chest into your chin and don't be afraid to use pillows to support your head or hips.

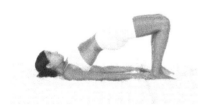

Seated Forward Bend Pose: also known as Paschimottanasana. If you have tight hamstrings you may need a strap, belt, tie, sash, etc. to assist you with this pose. Sitting with your legs out in front of you pull the fleshy part of each buttock away from you. Flex your feet with heels down and toes pointed towards the sky. Slowly reach your hands up toward the sky and bend forward reaching out keeping your back straight. Slowly bend forward grabbing the soles of your feet. If you cannot reach your toes place the strap around the bottom of your feet and pull yourself forward. Let your head hang and take nice deep breaths and then slowly roll yourself up to a seated position. If you have suffer from acute back pain or sciatica inflammation use caution with this pose.

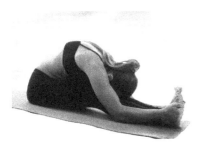

Bound Angle Pose: also known as Baddha Konasana or the Cobbler's Pose. While sitting with your legs out in front of you, bend your knees and bring your feet into what is known as a butterfly position. The bottom of your feet should be touching and your toes pointed out. The goal is bring your feet in as close as possible to your body but start off at position that is comfortable for you. With your hands grab the insides of your feet (arches) and slowly open them by rolling them out. As you do this your hips and knees will drop. Sit up as straight as possible and let yourself fall forward. Slowly round your back and shoulders forward letting everything fall. You can rest your rest your elbows on the inside of your knees to help open up your hips. Slowly roll up and repeat.

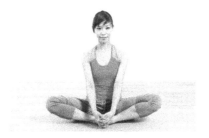

Wide Angle Seated Forward Bend Pose: also known as Upavistha Konasana.

In a sitting position extend of your legs out and away until they are in a wide V. Bring your arms straight up and over your head, bend from the hip and come forward and down as far as you can go.

Keep your toes pointing towards the sky. You can stay where you are or if you have a lot of flexibility you can grab the outer edges of your feet and bring the front of your spine and forehead all the way to the floor. Hold this pose for 15 to 20 seconds before returning to an upright position.

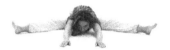

Seated Twist: called Ardha matsyendrasana in Sanskrit, is performed while sitting. Extend your legs while on the floor, and cross your left foot over your right thigh. This is when you should bend your right knee but be sure to keep your left knee positioned towards the ceiling. With your left hand behind you on the floor for stability, position your right elbow just outside of your left knee. Slowly begin to twist to the left while moving your abdomen, twist as far as you feel comfortable. Keep your rear firmly on the floor and repeat this exercise for both sides of your body.

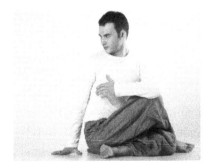

Child's Pose: also known as Balasana, is really good for letting you relax and breathe while on your back. Sit straight and rest on your heels. Roll your torso forward while you bring your forehead gently to the floor in front of your body. Stretch your arms out in front of you while lowering your chest to your knees. Maintain this position and exhale to position yourself deeper into the pose.

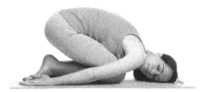

Legs Up The Wall Pose: also known as Viparita Karani, is beneficial for easing minor backaches and tired legs or feet. Lay on your back with your arms out away from your sides or above your head, whichever is most comfortable. Slowly lift your legs to a vertical position. Your legs and torso should resemble an "L" shape. Straighten your legs out as much as you can. Allow the weight of your thighs and belly to relax into your torso and then towards the back of your pelvis. Let your head lay naturally and enjoy this pose for 5 to 15 minutes while remembering to breathe.

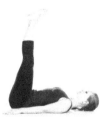

These Yoga poses improve flexibility. Often, the name of the pose will reflect on the visual appearance of the pose. To better understand and perform these poses, images have been provided with each pose to show you the correct positioning.

CHAPTER 8: QUICK TIPS ON HAVING A GREAT WORKOUT

We all should be working out. It does not matter where this takes place, either at your home in a designated area, or in a formal gym, maybe walking, doing dancercise, riding a bicycle, swimming or doing some gardening. It does not matter what takes place, the fact is we should keep moving. The best attitude to have is to exercise at least once per day and importantly, doing something you enjoy. The first quick tip to bear in mind is: If exercise is a big chore, then it will never take place. Should you be unable to work out every day, then a few times a week will be ideal.

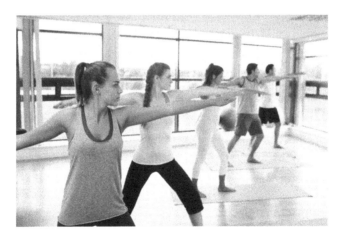

The second quick tip is: Create a positive mind set for your workout on a regular basis, as this is important for your body. Bodies are like machines, if they are not used they will shut down eventually. A fitness regime is essential to wellness so is a healthy and well balanced diet. They both go together to prolong life, at the same time allowing one to function properly by adding to your brain power which will enhance one's progress in the workplace. Regular exercise also improves attitudes when coping with the ups and downs in life. Bearing all this in mind, frequent work outs do more good than harm.

Another quick tip is: Do not start a work out by doing something difficult. Many beginners enthusiastically go to the gym and commence using machines that often harm them; in particular lifting weights that are far too heavy. There are instructors in most reputable gyms where you do not have to pay extra to get their advice. This service is offered free to all beginners, if it is not, and then look for another gym where you can talk with someone about what is best for your body type. An alternative is doing some research on the machines before trying them out. This can save a lot of discomfort and pain.

A quick tip to bear in mind is: Should your body have any old injuries you need to exercise with great caution, as the last thing that anyone wants is getting new injuries on top of ones that already exist. If you are using a home gym, this is just as important as working out in an established facility. One quick tip is: If you can afford to do so, get a personal trainer. This person does not have to work with you for a lifetime, but many personal trainers will give a reasonable quote for a one to three month time period to teach the best methods for working out, and what is needed to get your body in shape.

Another important tip to bear in mind is: Exercises are age appropriate. Now some people over 60 years old are able to exercise like a 30 year old person. This is not the case for most people, and in fact it is advisable not to over work your tendons and muscles as this can cause damage to the body. There are many resources that speak to this problem. Be careful that excessive strain is not placed on your body as you work out. Not all pain brings gain.

MEET THE AUTHOR

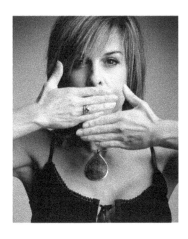

Author and healer Stacy Milescu leads her life toward peace and wellness. She has years of experience in the areas of spiritual healing, holistic health, yoga, and meditation. Through these disciplines, she is able to help people work through seasons of stress, grief, or injury, and also to find clarity and drive during more comfortable times.

Stacy first encountered yoga and meditation in 2004. She found herself nearly overwhelmed by anxiety while her husband was fighting cancer, and a friend suggested yoga as an option for centering herself. She quickly became interested in meditation and holistic health as well. With the help of a spiritual advisor and a fantastic yoga instruction, she regained her breath and survived those scary years. Now she and her husband—cancer free for almost 8 years now—do yoga together a couple times a week!

When she is not pursuing wellness, Stacy is generally enjoying time with her fantastic husband Gabe and their two boys Jake and Evan. As a family, they enjoy playing card games. She tends to lose at Euchre, but wins at Poker. She likes to think her penchant for serenity helps her poker face.

MORE BOOKS BY STACY MILESCU

Spiritual Healing Guide: How To Heal Yourself And Other Using Spiritual Methods